CARNITINE DEFICIENCY NUTRITION

Complete Guide To Understanding And Improving Health With Nutrition, Diagnosis, And Lifestyle

Dr. Holmgren Alfred

Carnitine Deficiency Nutrition: With Expert Guidance" is a comprehensive exploration of the critical role that carnitine plays in the human body and the consequences of its deficiency. From delving into the intricate biochemistry of carnitine to elucidating the various causes and types of deficiencies, this book serves as a beacon of knowledge for both professionals and individuals seeking to understand and address this nutritional concern. The multifaceted nature of carnitine deficiency, from physical symptoms to cognitive effects and long-term health implications, is thoroughly examined, providing a holistic perspective. Understanding carnitine and its physiological functions is paramount, as adequate levels are vital for optimal health. Through expert insights, readers gain a deep appreciation for the significance of maintaining proper carnitine levels and the potential consequences associated with deficiency. Furthermore, the book offers invaluable guidance on diagnosis, screening, and management strategies. Through detailed discussions on laboratory tests, differential diagnoses, and treatment options, readers are equipped with the knowledge necessary for effective intervention. Nutritional strategies, pharmacological interventions, and lifestyle modifications are meticulously explored, providing a comprehensive approach to addressing carnitine deficiency from various angles. Carnitine deficiency management is nuanced, with special considerations for different populations, including infants, pregnant women, and the elderly.

Practical recommendations for dietary planning, meal preparation, and supplementation enable readers to take proactive steps toward optimizing their carnitine levels and overall well-being.

Beyond immediate management, the book delves into future directions and research trends, shedding light on emerging therapies and their potential implications for public health policy. By staying up to date on the most recent advancements in carnitine research, readers can make informed decisions that benefit their own and others' health.

In summary, "Carnitine Deficiency Nutrition: With Expert Guidance" is more than just an instructional resource; it serves as a beacon of enlightenment and empowerment for individuals and professionals alike who want to battle carnitine insufficiency and enhance overall health.

Any resemblance to real events, places, or people—living or dead—is coincidental.

Disclaimer

This book, "Carnitine Deficiency Nutrition: With Expert Guidance," is intended for informational purposes only.

The information provided within this book is not intended to be a substitute for professional medical advice, diagnosis, or treatment. If you have any questions about a medical condition, always consult with your doctor or other qualified health provider.

The author of this book, [Your Name], is not a medical professional, and the content is based on research, personal experience, and expert opinions at the time of writing. However, medical knowledge and best practices are constantly changing, so the information in this book may become outdated or inaccurate over time.

The author does not promote any of the individuals, goods, websites, organizations, or other entities mentioned or referred to in this book; any references or mentions are solely for informational purposes and do not constitute an endorsement.

Readers are encouraged to independently verify any information provided in this book and consult with appropriate medical professionals before making any decisions regarding their health or nutrition regimen. The author and publisher of this book disclaim any liability or responsibility for any adverse consequences resulting directly or indirectly from the use or application of any information contained in this book.

By reading this book, you recognize and accept the conditions of this disclaimer.

INTRODUCTION

Carnitine deficiency is a metabolic disorder that can have profound consequences for human health and well-being. Carnitine, a naturally occurring compound synthesized in the body from the essential amino acid's lysine and methionine, plays a crucial role in energy metabolism by facilitating the transport of fatty acids into the mitochondria, where they undergo beta-oxidation to produce ATP, the body's primary energy currency.

Understanding Carnitine's Role In The Body

Carnitine is primarily known for its pivotal role in fatty acid metabolism, where it acts as a shuttle for transporting long-chain fatty acids into the mitochondria, the cellular powerhouses responsible for ATP production.

This process is essential for energy generation, particularly during periods of prolonged physical activity or fasting when glucose reserves become depleted and the body relies more heavily on fatty acid oxidation for fuel. In addition to its role

The Importance Of Adequate Carnitine Levels

Carnitine deficiency can cause impaired energy production, muscle weakness, fatigue, and cardiomyopathy, a condition characterized by abnormal heart muscle function. Adequate carnitine levels ensure efficient fatty acid oxidation, which is essential for meeting the energy demands of various tissues, particularly the heart and skeletal muscles. Additionally, carnitine

Carnitine deficiency can be caused by a variety of factors, including inadequate dietary intake, impaired biosynthesis, increased renal excretion, or genetic defects affecting carnitine transporters or biosynthetic enzymes. Primary carnitine deficiency, caused by genetic mutations affecting the OCTN2 transporter, results in impaired carnitine uptake by cells and can lead to severe metabolic complications such as muscle weakness, cardiomyopathy, and hypoglycemia. Secondary carnitine

carnitine deficiency is a metabolic disorder with significant implications for human health and well-being. Understanding the role of carnitine in energy metabolism and cellular homeostasis is essential for recognizing the importance of maintaining adequate carnitine levels. Carnitine deficiency patients can effectively manage their condition and improve their overall health through proper nutrition, accurate diagnosis, and lifestyle modifications.

CHAPTER 1
THE PHYSIOLOGY OF CARNITINE

Carnitine is an essential nutrient that plays a crucial role in energy metabolism within the human body. Its physiology revolves around facilitating the transport of long-chain fatty acids into the mitochondria, the powerhouse of cells, where they undergo beta-oxidation to produce energy. This process is vital for maintaining various physiological functions, particularly those with high energy demands, such as skeletal and cardiac muscles.

Carnitine's biochemistry includes its synthesis, metabolism, and biochemical reactions within the body. The amino acids lysine and methionine, as well as cofactors like vitamin C, iron, and certain enzymes, are used to produce both L-carnitine and acetyl-L-carnitine, which are then circulated to various tissues. Once inside the cells, carnitine undergoes enzymatic reactions.

Carnitine can be obtained through dietary sources or synthesized endogenously within the body. Dietary carnitine is primarily derived from animal products such as meat, poultry, fish, and dairy, with red meat being one of the richest sources. In contrast, plant-based foods generally contain lower levels of carnitine. Absorption of dietary carnitine occurs mainly in the small intestine, facilitated by active transport mechanisms. However, the efficiency of absorption varies among individuals and can be influenced by factors such as dietary composition and gut microbiota. Endogenous synthesis of carnitine primarily occurs in the liver and kidneys, starting from the precursor amino acids lysine and methionine. This process involves several enzymatic steps and requires cofactors such as iron, vitamin C, and certain B vitamins. The rate of endogenous carnitine synthesis is influenced by dietary intake, metabolic demands, and hormonal regulation. Despite the body's ability to synthesize carnitine, dietary intake remains crucial, particularly for individuals with specific dietary restrictions or conditions that may impair endogenous synthesis.

Transportation And Metabolism Of Carnitine In The Body

The transport and metabolism of carnitine in the body are tightly regulated processes essential for maintaining cellular energy homeostasis. Carnitine enters the bloodstream after absorption in the small intestine or release from tissue stores, where it is bound to plasma proteins for transport to various tissues.

The uptake of carnitine into cells is mediated by specific transporters located in the plasma membrane, such as OCTN2 (organic cation/carnitine transporter 2). Once inside the cell, carnitine is distributed to different cellular compartments, including the cytoplasm and mitochondria, to fulfill its metabolic functions. Within the mitochondria, carnitine plays a critical role in the transport of long-chain fatty acids across the inner mitochondrial membrane, a process necessary for beta-oxidation and ATP production. This transport process involves the carnitine shuttle system, which utilizes carnitine acyltransferases and carnitine translocase enzymes to facilitate the movement of fatty acids coupled with carnitine molecules.

Carnitine also serves as a cofactor for various enzymes involved in fatty acid metabolism, including carnitine palmitoyl transferases and carnitine acylcarnitine translocase. Moreover, carnitine participates in the regulation of metabolic pathways through its interaction with key metabolites, such as acyl-CoA derivatives, to maintain cellular energy balance and prevent the accumulation of toxic intermediates. Overall, the transport and metabolism of carnitine are tightly regulated processes essential for cellular energy metabolism and overall physiological function.

CHAPTER 2
CAUSES AND TYPES OF CARNITINE DEFICIENCY

Carnitine deficiency, a condition characterized by insufficient levels of carnitine in the body, can arise from a variety of causes, leading to significant implications for overall health and well-being. Understanding the factors contributing to carnitine deficiency is critical for effective diagnosis, treatment, and management. This deficiency can be broadly classified into two types: primary and secondary carnitine deficiency.

Individuals with primary carnitine deficiency frequently exhibit symptoms early in life, such as muscle weakness, hypoglycemia, cardiomyopathy, and metabolic disturbances. This genetic disorder inhibits the body's ability to produce or use carnitine effectively, resulting in decreased levels in tissues and systemic carnitine deficiency. The most common cause of primary carnitine deficiency is genetic mutations that affect carnitine biosynthesis or transportation.

Secondary carnitine deficiency, on the other hand, arises from acquired causes and underlying medical conditions that interfere with carnitine metabolism or increase its excretion. Various factors can contribute to secondary carnitine deficiency, including chronic diseases, certain medications, dietary deficiencies, and metabolic disorders. For instance, chronic kidney disease can impair renal reabsorption of carnitine, resulting in its loss in urine and subsequent

Several risk factors increase the likelihood of developing carnitine deficiency, irrespective of its primary or secondary nature. Genetic predisposition plays a significant role in primary carnitine deficiency, with mutations in genes involved in carnitine metabolism contributing to its development. Additionally, certain populations, such as infants and young children, are at higher risk due to increased metabolic demands and limited dietary intake. Individuals with chronic medical conditions, particularly those affecting the kidneys or liver, are also predisposed to secondary carnitine deficiency due to impaired metabolism or excretion of carnitine. Moreover, individuals following restrictive diets, such as vegans or vegetarians, may have reduced carnitine intake from food sources, further increasing their susceptibility to deficiency. Other risk factors include certain medications, such as antibiotics and antiretrovirals, which can interfere with carnitine absorption or metabolism, as well as intense physical activity or exercise, which may increase carnitine utilization.

carnitine deficiency encompasses a spectrum of conditions characterized by insufficient levels of carnitine in the body, with primary and secondary forms distinguished by their underlying causes. Primary carnitine deficiency results from genetic mutations that affect carnitine biosynthesis or transportation, while secondary carnitine deficiency arises from acquired causes such as chronic diseases, medications, and dietary deficiencies. Understanding the causes and risks

CHAPTER 3

SYMPTOMS AND CLINICAL MANIFESTATIONS

Physical Symptoms Of Carnitine Deficiency:

Carnitine deficiency, a condition characterized by inadequate levels of carnitine in the body, can manifest through a variety of physical symptoms. Carnitine plays a crucial role in energy metabolism, particularly in facilitating the transport of fatty acids into the mitochondria for oxidation. Thus, one of the primary physical symptoms of carnitine deficiency is fatigue and muscle weakness.

Furthermore, individuals with carnitine deficiency may experience cardiovascular symptoms such as chest pain (angina), palpitations, and cardiac arrhythmias. Carnitine is involved in maintaining the balance of fatty acids in the heart muscle, and its deficiency can impair cardiac function, potentially leading to serious complications. Additionally, muscle cramps and myalgias may result from carnitine deficiency, as muscles rely on adequate carnitine levels for optimal energy.

In severe cases, carnitine deficiency can cause skeletal muscle weakness and myopathy, exacerbating physical symptoms. Furthermore, individuals with carnitine deficiency may exhibit symptoms of hypoglycemia due to impaired fatty acid oxidation, as fatty acids serve as an important energy source during periods of fasting or low glucose availability.

These physical symptoms highlight the critical role of carnitine in various physiological processes.

Cognitive And Neurological Impacts:

Carnitine, in addition to its role in energy metabolism, has a significant impact on cognitive and neurological function. Carnitine deficiency can result in cognitive impairments such as memory loss, difficulty concentrating, and mental fatigue.

The brain relies on fatty acids as a major energy source, especially during periods of high metabolic demand or stress. Insufficient carnitine levels compromise the brain's ability to efficiently utilize fatty acids, potentially

Furthermore, carnitine deficiency has been associated with neurological symptoms including neuropathy, seizures, and encephalopathy. The nervous system is highly dependent on mitochondrial function and energy metabolism for proper functioning, and insufficient carnitine availability impairs the transport of fatty acids into the mitochondria, disrupting energy production and compromising neuronal integrity. As a result, individuals with carnitine deficiency may experience sensory

Furthermore, carnitine plays a critical role in neuroprotection and antioxidant defense mechanisms within the brain, and its deficiency may exacerbate oxidative stress and neuroinflammation, contributing to neuronal damage and neurodegenerative processes. Thus, addressing carnitine deficiency is essential not only for alleviating cognitive and neurological symptoms but also for preserving brain health and lowering the risk of neurodegenerative diseases in the long run.

Long-Term Health Consequences:

Untreated carnitine deficiency can have serious long-term health consequences, affecting multiple organ systems and increasing the risk of chronic diseases. Prolonged deficiency can lead to cardiomyopathy, a condition characterized by structural and functional abnormalities in the heart muscle, eventually resulting in heart failure and cardiovascular complications. Cardiomyopathy caused by carnitine deficiency is frequently associated with impaired energy metabolism, oxidative

Moreover, carnitine deficiency has been implicated in the development of metabolic disorders such as insulin resistance, obesity, and dyslipidemia. Carnitine plays a key role in regulating lipid metabolism and mitochondrial function, and its deficiency can disrupt these processes, leading to abnormal lipid accumulation, insulin signaling dysfunction, and metabolic imbalances. As a result, individuals with carnitine deficiency may be at an increased risk of developing type

Furthermore, carnitine deficiency can compromise immune function and predispose individuals to infections and inflammatory conditions. Carnitine is involved in modulating immune cell activity, cytokine production, and inflammatory responses, and its deficiency may impair immune surveillance and host defense mechanisms. Oxidative stress and mitochondrial dysfunction can exacerbate inflammation and tissue damage, contributing to

 Overall, recognizing the long-term health consequences of carnitine deficiency emphasizes the importance of proactive screening, diagnosis, and management strategies to prevent complications and optimize health outcomes. Addressing carnitine deficiency through nutritional interventions, supplementation, and lifestyle modifications can reduce the risk of developing chronic diseases and improve overall well-being.

CHAPTER 4
DIAGNOSIS AND SCREENING

Diagnosing and screening for carnitine deficiency is critical for identifying individuals at risk and initiating appropriate interventions to improve health outcomes. Carnitine deficiency is diagnosed using a variety of methods, including laboratory tests, clinical assessments, and screening protocols. Early detection and accurate diagnosis are essential for implementing targeted treatment strategies and preventing potential complications.

Laboratory Tests For Carnitine Levels:

Carnitine deficiency is diagnosed through laboratory tests that measure carnitine levels in blood, urine, or tissues. Quantitative methods like high-performance liquid chromatography (HPLC) or tandem mass spectrometry (LC-MS/MS) are commonly used to assess serum carnitine levels. These techniques provide accurate measurements of free carnitine (FC), acylcarnitine (AC), and total carnitine (TC) concentrations, allowing healthcare professionals to evaluate car

Differential Diagnosis For Carnitine Deficiency:

Primary carnitine deficiency is caused by genetic mutations that affect the carnitine transporter system, resulting in impaired carnitine uptake by cells. On the other hand, secondary carnitine deficiency can be caused by a variety of factors, including inadequate dietary intake, gastrointestinal disorders, renal dysfunction,

Screening Recommendations And Protocols:

Screening for carnitine deficiency is recommended for specific populations at increased risk, such as individuals with metabolic disorders, genetic predispositions, or chronic medical conditions affecting carnitine metabolism. Screening protocols may include targeted laboratory testing, clinical evaluations, and assessment of dietary habits and lifestyle factors. In some regions, newborn screening programs include carnitine deficiency as part of routine metabolic screening.

Carnitine deficiency diagnosis and screening require a multifaceted approach that includes laboratory testing, differential diagnosis considerations, and adherence to screening recommendations and protocols. Early detection and intervention are critical in optimizing health outcomes and preventing potential complications associated with carnitine deficiency.

CHAPTER 5
TREATMENT AND MANAGEMENT

Carnitine deficiency is a significant challenge in clinical practice, often necessitating a multifaceted approach to treatment and management. This deficiency can lead to various physiological disturbances, such as impaired fatty acid metabolism and energy production. Effective management strategies aim to address the underlying cause of deficiency, replenish carnitine levels, and optimize overall health outcomes.

Nutritional Strategies for Carnitine Repletion

Carnitine is primarily obtained through dietary sources, so ensuring adequate intake of carnitine-rich foods is essential. Among the richest natural sources of carnitine are red meat, poultry, fish, and dairy products. While vegetarians and vegans may have lower carnitine intake, plant-based sources such as avocados, asparagus, and whole grains can still contribute.

L-carnitine, the biologically active form of carnitine, is widely available as a dietary supplement, and supplementation doses may vary depending on the severity of the deficiency and individual response. To avoid overdosing or underdosing, blood carnitine levels must be monitored and supplementation adjusted accordingly.

Pharmacological interventions include supplements and medications.

To effectively manage carnitine deficiency, pharmacological interventions can be used in addition to dietary strategies. The primary pharmacological approach is L-carnitine supplementation, which is available in a variety of forms including oral capsules, liquid solutions, and intravenous formulations. These supplements aim to replenish carnitine stores, improve fatty acid metabolism, and increase energy production.

Aside from L-carnitine, certain medications can also affect carnitine levels. For example, valproic acid, which is used to treat epilepsy, can cause carnitine depletion through increased renal excretion. In such cases, L-carnitine supplementation may be required to mitigate the negative effects of medication-induced carnitine deficiency.

Lifestyle Changes to Improve Carnitine Levels

Regular physical activity promotes mitochondrial function and fatty acid oxidation, both of which rely on adequate carnitine levels for optimal performance. Lifestyle changes, in addition to dietary and pharmacological interventions, play an important role in supporting carnitine levels and overall health. Incorporating regular exercise into daily routines can help improve carnitine utilization and reduce the risk of deficiency.

Furthermore, managing stress levels and ensuring adequate sleep are important lifestyle factors that can impact carnitine metabolism. Chronic stress and sleep deprivation can disrupt metabolic processes, including carnitine synthesis and utilization. Implementing stress-reduction techniques such as mindfulness meditation, yoga, or relaxation exercises can help support carnitine homeostasis and improve overall well-being.

addressing carnitine deficiency requires a comprehensive approach that includes nutritional strategies, pharmacological interventions, and lifestyle modifications.

By optimizing carnitine intake, supplementing as needed, and adopting healthy lifestyle habits, individuals can effectively manage carnitine deficiency and promote optimal health outcomes.

CHAPTER 6
CARNITINE IN SPECIAL POPULATIONS

Carnitine, a compound synthesized in the liver and kidneys, plays a crucial role in energy metabolism by facilitating the transport of long-chain fatty acids into the mitochondria for beta-oxidation. However, deficiencies in carnitine can occur due to a variety of factors, leading to disruptions in energy production and potentially impacting overall health. Understanding the implications of carnitine deficiency in different populations, including infants and children, pregnancy,

Carnitine deficiency in infants and children can have profound effects on growth, development, and overall health. Neonatal carnitine deficiency may manifest shortly after birth, resulting in symptoms such as hypoglycemia, hepatomegaly, cardiomyopathy, and muscle weakness, which can be severe and life-threatening if left untreated. Additionally, children with certain metabolic disorders or chronic medical conditions may be at increased risk of developing carnet.

Insufficient carnitine levels during pregnancy may contribute to complications such as intrauterine growth restriction, preterm birth, and low birth weight, as maternal carnitine levels can impact fetal development and pregnancy outcomes. Additionally, carnitine plays an important role in placental function and fetal growth by facilitating the transfer of fatty acids across the placental barrier.

Elderly individuals are another population vulnerable to carnitine deficiency due to age-related changes in metabolism and nutrient absorption.

Age-related declines in carnitine levels have been observed in various tissues, including skeletal muscle and cardiac tissue, which can impair mitochondrial function and energy metabolism. Additionally, comorbidities commonly seen in older adults, such as cardiovascular disease, diabetes, and chronic kidney disease, may further exacerbate carnitine deficiency through increased metabolic demands or impaired renal clearance of carnitine. Consequently, elderly individuals may experience symptoms such as fatigue, muscle weakness, and exercise intolerance, which can negatively impact quality of life and functional independence. Strategies to address carnitine deficiency in the elderly may include dietary modifications, supplementation, and lifestyle interventions aimed at optimizing nutrient intake, promoting physical activity, and managing underlying health conditions.

carnitine deficiency can have significant implications for health and well-being across various population groups, including infants and children, pregnant women, and the elderly. Recognizing the unique considerations and challenges associated with carnitine deficiency in these populations is essential for early detection, intervention, and prevention of associated health complications. Addressing carnitine deficiency through targeted nutrition

CHAPTER 7
DIETARY RECOMMENDATIONS & MEAL PLANNING

Carnitine deficiency can cause a variety of health issues due to its role in energy metabolism and the transport of fatty acids into mitochondria for β-oxidation.

To ensure adequate intake of this essential nutrient while maintaining a balanced diet, meal planning for those with carnitine deficiency should focus on incorporating foods rich in carnitine.

Carnitine-Rich Foods And Sources:

Identifying carnitine-rich foods and food sources is crucial for individuals with carnitine deficiency to address their nutritional needs effectively. Animal-based products are among the primary sources of carnitine, with red meat, poultry, and fish containing relatively high concentrations. For example, a 3-ounce serving of cooked beef provides approximately 81 milligrams of carnitine, while chicken breast contains about 3-5 milligrams per ounce. Additionally, dairy

Sample meal plans for carnitine deficiency:

Creating sample meal plans for people with carnitine deficiency can help ensure adequate nutrient intake while promoting dietary variety and adherence. A balanced meal plan for someone with carnitine deficiency may include a combination of lean protein sources, healthy fats, complex carbohydrates, and plenty of fruits and vegetables. For breakfast, options might include a spinach and mushroom omelette with whole-grain toast and sliced avocado.

Grilling, baking, or steaming can help preserve the carnitine content of meats and vegetables while minimizing added fats and oils. Marinating meats in citrus-based or vinegar-based sauces before cooking can also enhance flavor without compromising nutritional integrity.

CHAPTER 8
NUTRITIONAL SUPPLEMENTS AND ADJUNCTIVE THERAPIES

Carnitine is a vital compound in the human body that plays a crucial role in energy metabolism, particularly in the transport of fatty acids into the mitochondria for oxidation. Carnitine deficiency can lead to a variety of health issues, including muscle weakness, fatigue, and cardiac abnormalities. Therefore, addressing carnitine deficiency often involves supplementation with carnitine, as well as adjunct therapies to support overall health and wellness.

An Overview Of Carnitine Supplements:

L-carnitine, the biologically active form of carnitine found in the body, is commonly used as a supplement to address deficiencies and support various health conditions. L-carnitine supplements are available in a variety of formulations, including oral capsules, liquid solutions, and intravenous injections. The dosage of carnitine supplementation varies depending on the severity of the deficiency.

Research suggests that carnitine supplementation may benefit individuals with carnitine deficiency, as well as those with certain medical conditions such as cardiovascular disease, diabetes, and muscle disorders. However, the efficacy of carnitine supplements in improving health outcomes remains a topic of debate, and more clinical studies are needed to reach definitive conclusions.

Supplementary Treatments for Carnitine Deficiency:

In addition to carnitine supplementation, complementary therapies like acupuncture and herbal therapy can help manage carnitine deficit and promote general health.

Dietary interventions aim to optimize nutrient intake to support carnitine metabolism and energy production. Carnitine-rich foods include meat, fish, poultry, and dairy products. Vegetarians and vegans may have lower carnitine levels due to dietary restrictions, requiring supplementation or dietary modifications.

Regular physical activity and stress management can have an impact on carnitine levels and overall health. Exercise promotes mitochondrial function and energy metabolism, which may help alleviate symptoms associated with carnitine deficiency. Meditation and yoga, for example, can support cellular energy production and improve overall well-being.

Alternative therapies like acupuncture and herbal medicine are often used in conjunction with conventional treatments to address carnitine deficiency and associated symptoms. While the evidence supporting their efficacy is limited, some individuals may find relief from symptoms through these modalities. It's essential to consult qualified healthcare professionals before integrating complementary therapies into a treatment regimen.

Safety And Efficacy Considerations:

While carnitine supplements are generally considered safe for most individuals when used as directed, adverse effects such as gastrointestinal discomfort and fishy body odor may occur, particularly at higher doses. When considering carnitine supplementation and adjunct therapies for carnitine deficiency, safety and efficacy are paramount.

Excessive carnitine intake has raised long-term safety concerns, including the possibility of cardiovascular complications and changes in endogenous carnitine synthesis. To avoid adverse effects, carnitine levels should be monitored regularly and supplementation adjusted accordingly.

Furthermore, the efficacy of carnitine supplementation in improving health outcomes remains uncertain, with conflicting evidence from clinical studies. While some research suggests potential benefits for specific medical conditions, more robust evidence is required to make definitive recommendations.

nutritional supplements and adjunct therapies play a crucial role in managing carnitine deficiency and promoting overall health. Carnitine supplementation, along with complementary therapies such as dietary interventions and lifestyle modifications, can help support energy metabolism and alleviate symptoms associated with carnitine deficiency. However, safety and efficacy considerations should be carefully evaluated, and individuals should consult healthcare.

CHAPTER 9

LIFESTYLE STRATEGIES FOR OPTIMAL CARNITINE LEVELS.

Carnitine, a compound synthesized from the amino acids lysine and methionine, plays a crucial role in energy metabolism by facilitating the transport of long-chain fatty acids into the mitochondria for oxidation. Lifestyle factors such as exercise, stress management, and sleep patterns all have an impact on carnitine levels and utilization.

Endurance training, in particular, has been shown to increase carnitine levels in skeletal muscle, which improves fat utilization and exercise performance. Regular physical activity promotes the synthesis of carnitine and enhances its transport into muscle cells, where it aids in the conversion of fatty acids into energy during prolonged or intense exercise.

Chronic stress can disrupt metabolic processes and deplete carnitine levels, leading to impaired energy production and increased susceptibility to fatigue. Stress-reduction strategies such as mindfulness meditation, deep breathing exercises, and progressive muscle relaxation can help mitigate stress's negative impact on carnitine metabolism.

Adequate sleep is essential for tissue restoration and repair, including the synthesis and replenishment of carnitine stores. Research has shown that sleep deprivation can disrupt carnitine metabolism and impair mitochondrial function, leading to decreased energy production and increased oxidative stress.

To summarize, adopting lifestyle strategies that prioritize exercise, stress management, and sleep hygiene is essential for maintaining optimal carnitine levels and supporting overall health and well-being. By incorporating regular physical activity, implementing stress-reduction techniques, and prioritizing adequate sleep and recovery practices, individuals can enhance carnitine metabolism, optimize energy production, and promote metabolic resilience.

CHAPTER 10
FUTURE DIRECTIONS AND RESEARCH TRENDS

Emerging Research on Carnitine and Health

Recent advancements in research have shed light on the multifaceted role of carnitine in health and disease. While historically known for its involvement in fatty acid metabolism and energy production, contemporary studies have unveiled its significance in various physiological processes, ranging from cardiovascular health to neurological function. Emerging research is exploring the intricate mechanisms underlying carnitine's actions, including its impact on mitochondrial function, cellular signaling pathways, and gene expression.

Moreover, investigations are delving into the potential therapeutic applications of carnitine in managing diverse health conditions, such as metabolic disorders, neurodegenerative diseases, and cardiovascular ailments. Novel insights into the role of carnitine in regulating metabolism, oxidative stress, and inflammation have sparked interest in developing targeted interventions to modulate carnitine levels for optimizing health outcomes. Furthermore, advancements in analytical techniques have facilitated the identification of biomarkers associated with carnitine deficiency, enabling early diagnosis and intervention strategies. Overall, the burgeoning field of carnitine research holds promise for uncovering novel therapeutic avenues and enhancing our understanding of its intricate interplay with human physiology.

Innovative Therapeutic Approaches.

The expanding understanding of carnitine's physiological functions has paved the way for innovative therapeutic approaches aimed at addressing carnitine deficiency and related health conditions.

Traditional interventions for carnitine deficiency have primarily focused on carnitine supplementation to restore intracellular carnitine levels and alleviate symptoms associated with impaired fatty acid metabolism.

However, recent advancements have diversified therapeutic strategies, including targeted drug development, gene therapy, and dietary interventions. Pharmacological agents targeting carnitine biosynthesis, transport mechanisms, and cellular uptake pathways are under investigation to enhance carnitine availability and efficacy in specific tissues. Gene therapy approaches leveraging gene editing technologies offer promising prospects for correcting genetic mutations underlying primary carnitine deficiency and related disorders.

Moreover, dietary interventions emphasizing carnitine-rich foods, such as red meat, fish, and dairy products, or supplementation with precursors like trimethyllysine, are being explored as adjunctive therapies to optimize carnitine status and metabolic function.

These innovative therapeutic approaches hold the potential for personalized management strategies tailored to individual needs and disease states, heralding a new era in the clinical management of carnitine deficiency and associated conditions.

Implications Of Public Health Policy

The growing recognition of carnitine's importance in health and disease has profound implications for public health policy and healthcare delivery.

Carnitine deficiency, whether primary or secondary, poses significant health risks and can lead to a spectrum of metabolic, neurological, and cardiovascular disorders. Therefore, integrating carnitine assessment into routine screening protocols and diagnostic algorithms holds promise for early detection and intervention, thus mitigating the burden of associated morbidity and mortality.

Furthermore, promoting awareness of carnitine-rich dietary sources and optimizing nutritional strategies can help prevent deficiencies and promote overall health and well-being.

Public health initiatives aimed at improving dietary diversity, promoting physical activity, and addressing socioeconomic disparities can contribute to reducing the prevalence of carnitine deficiency and its associated comorbidities on a population level. Additionally, fostering interdisciplinary collaborations between healthcare professionals, researchers, policymakers, and community stakeholders is essential for developing evidence-based guidelines, implementing preventive measures, and optimizing healthcare delivery for individuals at risk of carnitine deficiency.

By prioritizing carnitine-related research, education, and policy initiatives, public health efforts can effectively address the burgeoning challenges posed by carnitine deficiency and enhance health outcomes across diverse populations.

CONCLUSION

carnitine deficiency represents a complex and multifaceted health concern with far-reaching implications for metabolism, cellular function, and overall well-being. While significant strides have been made in elucidating the physiological roles of carnitine and its involvement in various disease states, much remains to be explored, particularly regarding its intricate interplay with genetic, environmental, and lifestyle factors. The integration of emerging research findings into clinical practice offers promising avenues for improving diagnostic accuracy, therapeutic efficacy, and preventive interventions for individuals at risk of carnitine deficiency. Innovative therapeutic approaches, informed by advances in pharmacology, genetics, and nutrition, hold the potential to revolutionize the management of carnitine-related disorders and enhance patient outcomes. Moreover, recognizing the broader implications of carnitine deficiency for public health policy underscores the importance of proactive measures to promote awareness, screening, and access to appropriate interventions on a population level.

By fostering collaborative efforts among researchers, healthcare providers, policymakers, and community stakeholders, we can address the multifaceted challenges posed by carnitine deficiency and pave the way toward a healthier future for all.